Natural Liver Flush

Natural Liver Flush

7-Day Liver Cleanse Diet to Revitalize Your Health, Detox Your Body, and Reverse Fatty Liver

Julia Grady

Dylanna Publishing

First edition: 2014

Disclaimer

This book is for informational purposes only. The views expressed are those of the author alone, and should not be taken as expert, legal, or medical advice. The reader is responsible for his or her own actions.

Every attempt has been made to verify the accuracy of the information in this publication. However, neither the author nor the publisher assumes any responsibility for errors, omissions, or contrary interpretation of the material contained herein.

This book is not intended to provide medical advice. Please see your health care professional before embarking on any new diet or exercise program. The reader should regularly consult a physician in matters relating to his/her health and particularly with respect to any symptoms that may require diagnosis or medical attention.

Table of Contents

Introduction

The liver is arguably the most important organ in the human body. Its health and proper functioning is vital to your overall health and well-being. Yet the stresses and toxins that are typical in a modern lifestyle are causing unprecedented strains on the liver and, some would say, an epidemic in health-related problems associated with an unhealthy liver.

Luckily, it is possible to detoxify your liver and return it to its peak functioning. This book will show you how you can flush your liver of toxins, detoxify your body, and restore yourself to peak health. The gentle, natural, 7-day plan will have you looking younger, feeling more energetic, and dropping pounds.

Why Should You Do a Liver Flush and Detoxification?

Nature has planned everything so precisely and the perfection of the human body is without question— from the macro level right down to the level of molecules and atoms, all the body's systems work in sync in an organized fashion. The body's ability to maintain homeostasis, or balance, is so flawless that reactions stop when they are supposed to, and start on their own. Why then do we need to concern ourselves with detoxification, shouldn't the body be able to handle this by itself?

In a perfect world, yes, it should. But, unfortunately, most of us do not live in a perfect world and so the liver needs a little help to remain in peak functioning.

The liver, being the metabolic center of the body, has been greatly affected by the stresses of modern living , which typically includes a poor diet and exposure to many environmental toxins. Some of the typical contaminants that can stress and overload the liver include:

* Sugar (including high-fructose corn syrup)

* Alcohol

* High-carbohydrate diet

* Caffeine

* Processed foods

* Medications (including anti-inflammatories such as acetaminophen)

* Environmental toxins (including pesticides, pollution, herbicides, cleaning products)

* Heavy metals (including lead, mercury, arsenic, aluminum—found in foods, dental fillings, etc.)

Exposure to all of these contaminants, which can be almost impossible to avoid, can overburden the liver, the organ responsible for processing toxins from the body. When the liver is overloaded, it can lead to a variety of health problems. Some symptoms of an overburdened liver include:

* Fatigue

* Poor sleep

* Brain fog, memory disturbances

* Muscle and joint pain

* Weight gain, especially around the abdomen (a spare tire appearance)

* Headaches

* Puffiness and dark circles under the eyes

* Sinus congestion

* Frequent colds and flus

* Sexual dysfunction

* Heartburn and indigestion

* Constipation and /or diarrhea

* Skin problems – dryness, rashes, itchiness, yellowing

* Canker sores

* Abdominal pain

* Loss of appetite

These are all signs and symptoms that your liver is not functioning as it should and is in need of help.

To understand the importance of the liver and how its dysfunction can lead to major health problems, such as fatty liver disease and its consequences, it is essential to understand the workings of the liver and its vital role in the human body.

What's So Special About the Liver?

While the skin is the largest organ overall, the liver is the largest internal organ and it maintains the title of being the largest gland in the body. Just like other organs, various metabolic functions are unique to the liver and cannot be fulfilled without it.

The Anatomy of the Liver

The liver, weighing approximately 3 1/2 lbs, is a reddish brown organ, located on the right side of the abdomen, and is normally protected by the ribcage and thus cannot be felt, unless it is markedly enlarged.

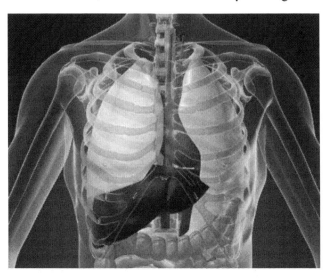

The normal liver has a vascular network of vessels and is of a firm consistency. It is divided histologically into two regions—the right and the left lobes. The right lobe is the larger of the two with no functional difference from the smaller left lobe. What makes the liver such a great detox agent is the rich vascular blood supply that spans the entire organ allowing the channel of arteries and veins greater surface area coverage when the blood passes through the liver for detoxification.

The Functions of the Liver

The liver plays a role in many of the vital functions of the human body including digestion, metabolism, and the immune system. One of the liver's main functions in the body is detoxification. It works by filtering the blood coming from the digestive tract and removing any toxins, such as alcohol and drugs, that enter the bloodstream with the digested nutrients.

The functions of the liver include:

> * **Detoxification.** It helps detoxify the noxious chemicals formed during regular metabolic activities of the body and serves as a natural detoxifier that continuously removes harmful substances.

* **Bile production**. The liver produces bile, which is an important agent in the digestion and emulsification of fats. It is the main glandular secretion that the liver synthesizes and is stored in the gall bladder, from where it is periodically released into the intestines.

* **Blood production**. The liver produces several components of blood plasma: albumins, prothrombin, and fibrinogen.

* **Conversion of toxins**. Ammonia is converted into urea by the liver.

* **Glucose**. One of the most important functions of the liver is conversion of blood sugar into glycogen. This is the key process that keeps the body going when there is no glucose intake. The stored glycogen is broken down into glucose when other sources of glucose are unavailable.

* **Storage of nutrients**. The liver also stores many vitamins, minerals, and other nutrients. Fatty acids are stored there along with vitamins A, D, E, K, and B12.

* **Blood clotting**. The liver is the major source of production of factors of the coagulation cascade that help form blood clots. Therefore, it is not uncommon to encounter bleeding disorders where liver function is compromised.

These are just some of the many functions performed by the liver. Let's take a moment now to understand how the liver works within the digestive process and how it processes the glucose it gets from the diet.

The moment we eat, our digestive system kicks off. It digests all the food we have eaten and subjects it to different enzymes that break it down into basic units that can be used by the body. This is how carbohydrates get converted into glucose—the main source of energy for the human body. The amount of sugar (glucose) that is needed by the body is taken up by the tissues, while the excess is converted to glycogen. The essential proteins get deposited or incorporated into the metabolic cycles or get converted to nitrogen and urea for excretion, while the fats are converted to fatty acids and are deposited in the fat cells.

These molecules (amino acids, fatty acids, and glucose) are then taken up by various receptors in the intestine and are placed in diverse cycles and areas of the body as they circulate in the blood. All this is part of the body's normal metabolism.

Liver Health and Disease

As we have shown, the liver is truly an amazing organ with many diverse functions. The liver is one of the most important organs in the human body and its proper functioning is vital to our overall health and well-being. Problems normally encountered with a diseased liver vary from benign courses of hepatic dysfunction to liver cancer and cirrhosis, both of which have a very poor prognosis.

The main types of liver disease are:

* Acute liver failure

* Alcoholic liver disease

* Alpha-1-antitrypsin deficiency

*Autoimmune hepatitis

*Bile duct obstruction

*Chronic liver failure

* Cirrhosis

* Enlarged liver

* Gilbert's syndrome

* Hemochromatosis

* Hepatitis A, B, C, D, E

* Liver adenoma

* Liver cancer

* Liver cyst

* Liver hemangioma

* Liver nodule (focal nodular hyperplasia)

* Nonalcoholic fatty liver disease

* Parasitic infection

* Portal vein thrombosis

* Primary biliary cirrhosis

* Toxic hepatitis

* Wilson's disease

One disease that is on the rise, almost to epidemic proportions, is fatty liver disease. That is the subject to which we now turn.

What Is Fatty Liver Disease?

A fatty liver is one in which there is a high accumulation of fat (over 10 percent). Fatty tissues that cause inflammation replace the normal structures of the liver. Usually inflammation is followed by repair that restores the typical function of the liver and regenerates the lost tissues. In this case, however, repeated insults to the liver causes faulty repair, so that instead of restoring the normal cells of the liver, fat is deposited instead.

In the course of fatty liver disease, there is a gradual decline in liver function that in the later stages causes increased symptoms. Early in the course of the disease, a person may not experience any symptoms at all. However, as time passes, the person may feel fatigued and may gain weight, or if she or he is already overweight or obese, may be unable to lose weight.

A fatty liver has a yellowish appearance and is usually swollen and enlarged due to excessive fat accumulation.

Normally, the liver has a bit of fat stored for functional purposes. When fat accumulation exceeds the normal amount that is typically present in the liver, there is a decline in the integrity of the organ. Liver function is compromised and as a result, it can no longer work as efficiently as it could before.

Healthy liver   Fatty liver

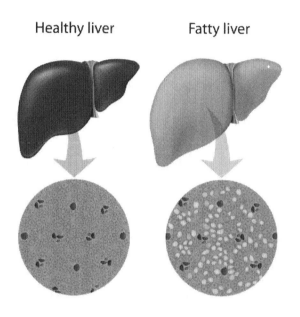

Causes and Prevalence

Statistical data obtained through various research studies show marked increase in liver disease. In surveys conducted during 1988-2008, prevalence of liver diseases, particularly non-alcoholic fatty liver disease, had risen from 5.51 percent to 11 percent, or a doubling of incidence of disease.

During the years 1988-1994, approximately 46.8 percent of liver disease was related to non-alcoholic fatty liver disease and this figure rose to 75.1 percent in the United States by 2006.

What is causing this increase?

Genetics plays an important role in the development of fatty liver. In addition, excessive alcohol consumption plays a major role. Lastly, a diet full of processed foods, sugars, and starches is implicated in the marked rise in fatty liver disease.

Genetics may be involved with how much alcohol consumption the liver can tolerate or if the enzymes available for the breakdown of alcohol are present—or if present, are functional. With permanent liver damage, the normal parts of the liver may get converted to scar tissue and the liver may become cirrhotic. This may lead to liver cancer or liver failure, both of which are usually fatal.

Types of Fatty Liver

Fatty liver disease can be classified into two types.

1. Alcoholic liver disease (ALD)
2. Non-alcoholic fatty liver disease (NAFLD)

We'll discuss both the diseases in detail, highlighting the causes and natural treatments available to help combat them.

Alcoholic Liver Disease

Alcoholic liver disease (ALD), as the name suggests, is one that is associated with excessive intake of alcohol. Alcohol abuse, along with causing a variety of neurological and psychological problems, renders the liver useless over time.

Excessive alcohol consumption is a major problem, not only among older people, but also among young adults. More than 15 million people in the United States either abuse or overuse alcohol and a large majority of them, perhaps even all of them, will likely develop a fatty liver.

The liver is the main organ that helps to clear alcohol from the body and, being the main site for alcohol metabolism, it is severely affected by both binge drinking and alcohol abuse. To understand how alcohol affects the liver, it is important to understand how its metabolism in the body occurs and how this is harmful.

The normal amount of alcohol that is generally considered safe for men is up to four drinks in one day, however the total number of drinks per week should not in any case exceed 14 drinks. For women, the safe amount is two drinks per day but not more than seven drinks in a week. These guidelines have been set by the National Institute on Alcohol Abuse and Alcoholism (NIAAA). A standard drink means a 12 ounce beer or 5 ounce glass wine or 1.5 ounce 80 proof liquor, respectively.

In addition, blood alcohol content, or BAC, should not exceed 0.08 at any time. How much a person can safely drink is influenced by body mass. The greater the mass, the greater the alcohol distribution and the lesser the BAC. Since the liver can only clear about one unit of alcohol per hour, it is recommended that the rate of alcohol intake should not exceed the rate that the liver can remove it.

Alcohol is considered a poison by the body and unlike the metabolic pathways of fats, carbohydrates, and proteins, there is no "natural" place for alcohol in our system. Even with consumption of limited amounts of alcohol, our body shuts off all the other processes and starts to clear this unwanted substance from the circulation. The most important enzymes in this process are the duo, *alcohol dehydrogenase* and *aldehyde dehydrogenase.*

Alcohol dehydrogenase converts ethanol, the alcohol consumed, into *acetaldehyde.* Researchers believe that the ethanol may not actually cause as many problems as the acetaldehyde. The acetaldehyde is an unwanted substance by our bodies and needs to be broken down as well. Although it does not remain in the system for that long, it still causes many unwanted effects. For starters, it is a known carcinogen and a highly toxic substance, and high levels in the liver renders the liver cells open to injury. Metabolism in tissues other than the liver, such as in the pancreas, also causes direct injury to these tissues.

To breakdown acetaldehyde, the body uses the enzyme aldehyde dehydrogenase, which converts it to acetic acid or vinegar. The acetic acid is then either taken up by various tissues (muscles, heart, kidneys) to be converted into carbon dioxide and water and eventually excreted out, or it can be converted to acetyl coenzyme A and subsequently converted to fatty acids.

Now, the liver only has a limited supply of these enzymes and during a period of high alcohol consumption, these enzymes are used up faster than they can be replenished. Therefore, the alcohol isn't cleared from the system as early as it normally is. So the time taken by the liver to clear the alcohol from the body increases, and all the while other vital processes remain halted while the liver exhausts itself trying to detoxify the body.

With the direct toxic effects of the acetaldehyde, the liver is no longer able to process the fats as it normally does in a healthy state. The result is a high level of circulating fat that accumulates in the liver and other organs causing functional impairment. Given an additional stressor, like an infection, the liver may not be able to cope with the added abuse and may develop scarring, known as *cirrhosis,* and this can eventually develop into liver failure or liver cancer.

Non-Alcoholic Fatty Liver Disease

Non-alcoholic fatty liver disease (NAFLD) is basically the same disease but occurs due to factors not related to alcohol consumption. In some cases, NAFLD may progress to nonalcoholic steatohepatitis or NASH.

In this case, the liver also undergoes massive depositions of fat, only with a different cause. While alcoholic fatty liver disease occurs due to excessive alcohol consumption, non-alcoholic fatty liver disease may be associated with an array of disorders that include obesity and other medical conditions such as high cholesterol, metabolic syndrome, or diabetes mellitus. It may arise due to some infection, either viral or bacterial, or it may be due to inflammation. Intake of drugs, including overuse of acetaminophen and ibuprofen, may also be a factor in the development of non-alcoholic fatty liver disease and NASH. In addition, genetics likely play a role.

A state of malnutrition, or rapid weight loss, may also lead to liver damage that could develop into fatty liver. Various types of systemic or autoimmune diseases may serve as a cause. There are many factors that could lead to the development of a fatty liver. However, diet has been shown to play a major causative role.

Many people believe that non-alcoholic fatty liver disease (NAFLD) is due to a high intake of fat. However, recent studies have revealed that a diet that is high in carbohydrates is the main culprit.

So how does fatty liver happen? Research shows that when people consume a high-carbohydrate diet, there is an excess of glucose circulating in the blood. The excess sugars undergo glycogenesis and are converted to glycogen. Part of the sugar molecules (glucose and fructose) get converted to triglycerides, which is a kind of fat, and this leads to a greater lipid production. This is especially true for fructose, which is only converted by the liver to glycogen in small amounts and into triglycerides in greater amounts. Hence high fructose corn syrup is one of the main culprits implicated in fatty liver disease.

With a high level of carbohydrates in the bloodstream, the pancreas releases insulin to help regulate the surplus. People who are diabetic or pre-diabetic, or have metabolic syndrome, are more at risk for developing fatty liver. This is because lack of insulin or insulin resistance causes high levels of circulating blood sugars that cannot be taken up by the tissues. The body cannot immediately use all of this extra glucose and so it gets stored as fat reserves. Some of these excess fat deposits get stored in the liver and consequently a fatty liver develops.

Risk Factors for Fatty Liver Disease

Here is a summary of the risk factors for developing both alcoholic and non-alcohol fatty liver disease.

* Excessive alcohol consumption

* Diet high in processed foods, including simple carbohydrates and high-fructose corn syrup

* Being overweight or obese

* Overuse of over-the-counter medications that are toxic to the liver, including acetaminophen and ibuprofen

* Having high cholesterol and/or high triglycerides

* Being diabetic or pre-diabetic

* Metabolic syndrome

* Rapid weight loss or malnutrition

* Hepatitis

Signs and Symptoms

Initially, there are typically not any symptoms of liver disease. Liver disease starts off without any outward signs and slowly creeps up, taking 10 years or more before any symptoms can be felt. And, when someone does experience symptoms, the damage is often far greater than expected. It is therefore of great importance, if liver disease is suspected, to have regular checkups to ensure proper liver function and integrity.

Some general symptoms of poor liver health include:

Fatigue. Feeling fatigued for no obvious reason. Feeling low and down. When the metabolic needs of the body are not met, the system slows down and fatigue is the result. Fatigue, however, is fairly common and not solely indicative of liver disease.

Weight loss or loss of appetite. This is another indicator that the liver may not be holding up as it should.

Nausea. Some people might experience nausea and vomiting due to liver dysfunction.

Brain fog. Trouble with concentration, memory or general confusion.

These early symptoms are all quite general and vague and could be associated with other problems besides the liver.

As the disease progresses, more advanced symptoms will appear:

Jaundice. A yellow appearance of the skin and eyes. This occurs due to failure of the liver to clear bilirubin from the blood.

Fluid retention. Around the abdomen or in the extremities such as ankles.

Pain. Pain may be felt in the upper right abdomen area.

Bleeding. People may also experience bleeding disorders since the liver is not functioning properly to produce the factors that help regulate and maintain homeostasis.

Diagnosis

People who suspect they have liver disease should first consult with their doctors. The symptoms of fatty liver can mimic those of other diseases and what a person might suspect to be a fatty liver might be another disease entirely or, in many cases, not a disease at all.

During a routine checkup a doctor may notice an enlarged liver during a physical exam. Blood tests are also used to diagnose fatty liver.

The *liver function tests (LFTs)* are a group of tests that evaluate the amount of liver enzymes that are present in the blood. If these enzymes are elevated, this indicates a problem, though it may not necessarily be fatty liver. If the enzymes are normal, we still cannot absolutely rule out the presence of fatty liver.

Imaging tests, such as ultrasound, CT scan, or an MRI, are also used in diagnosis. These show the structure of the liver and can give a more accurate picture of fatty deposits and the extent of the damage.

Finally, a *liver biopsy* is the only sure way to confirm the diagnosis and extent of liver disease. This is usually only done after other tests have indicated a problem.

If you suspect you have, or have been diagnosed with fatty liver disease, don't despair. In the large majority of cases, fatty liver can be stopped and reversed and the liver will regenerate itself back to health. Read on to find out about how the 7-day liver flush cleanse can jump start your liver's detoxification as well supplements to take and changes you can make in your overall diet to support a healthy liver.

Diet and Lifestyle Changes to Support Liver Health

There are many ways you can improve your liver health and reverse fatty liver disease. Top among these is your diet.

Eating habits play a key role in the development of fatty liver and the standard American diet (SAD) is extremely hard on the liver. The typical person consumes an abundance of processed foods, fast foods, high-fat foods, sugar, and simple carbohydrates. In order to stop and reverse the damage to your liver, there are certain lifestyle changes you are going to need to make. While these may seem difficult at first, you will find the benefits far outweigh the sacrifices.

Foods to Avoid

Carbohydrates. Here we are talking about simple carbohydrates found in white sugar, white flour, and most processed foods. These foods also tend to contain high-fructose corn syrup. These foods put a strain on your liver due to their high glucose content. The liver cannot handle a flood of glucose hitting it all at once and so much of simple carbohydrates get turned into fat.

Saturated fats. Although carbohydrates are the key component that leads to a fatty liver, saturated fats certainly do not help. Most processed and fast foods contain this type of fat. Eliminate saturated fats and trans fats from your diet and replace them with the healthy fats found in foods such as olive oil, avocado, coconut oil, and nuts.

Sugar. An excess of sugar is damaging to the liver. Try and avoid foods that contain added sugar.

Caffeine. Too much caffeine is not good for your liver. Limit the amount of coffee you consume each day. Avoid colas and energy drinks which are high in caffeine and sugar.

Foods that Support a Healthy Liver

Now that we've outlined those things that should be avoided, it's time to focus on the foods that can help decrease your risk of liver-related health problems.

Fruits. Full of vitamins, minerals, and fiber, these are an essential part of the diet. It is best to consume fruit in its whole form rather than as juice. Berries and citrus fruits are great choices for liver health.

Vegetables. Vegetables are full of fiber, antioxidants, and vitamins. The majority of your diet should be made up of vegetables. Aim for at least 5 and up to 10 servings a day. Variety is key here, so be sure to include dark leafy greens and cruciferous vegetables, as well as yellow, orange, and red vegetables. Eat them raw for the most dense nutrients.

Whole grains. Avoid refined, white grains and flour. Instead choose whole wheat, oats, brown rice, and quinoa. These provided the necessary fiber, release glucose slower, and will provide a steady source of energy.

Lean meat and protein. Protein is the building block of our bodies. Choose lean cuts of beef, chicken, turkey, pork, and fish. Grass-fed, hormone-free meat is ideal. Other good sources of protein are legumes, eggs, tofu, nuts, and seeds.

Healthy fats. Having a fatty liver does not mean you should avoid all fats. While saturated and trans fats are best avoided, healthy unsaturated fats should be a part of your diet. Good sources of these are olive oil, flaxseed oil, coconut oil, fish oil, avocados, and nuts and seeds.

Water. Water is essential for helping the liver clear itself and the body of harmful toxins. Make water your go-to beverage of choice. If you don't like the taste of plain water, you can add a squeeze of fresh lemon or lime.

Lifestyle Changes for Liver Health

In addition to diet, there are other lifestyle changes that can improve your liver health.

Reduce or Eliminate Alcohol. As already discussed, alcohol is quite destructive to the liver and is best avoided. Drinking in moderation is okay, but you should abstain entirely for a period of at least 30 days to allow time for your liver to replenish itself.

Over-the-counter medications. All substances that enter your body, including medications, are processed through the liver. One that is known to be particularly harmful to the liver is acetaminophen (Tylenol). Try to limit the intake of acetaminophen as much as possible and do not take it if you consume alcohol. The combination of the two can cause serious damage to your liver.

Quit Smoking. Although the greatest problems seen with smoking are related to the lungs and the heart, the liver is also damaged due to the direct harmful effects of the toxins circulating in the blood.

Control Your Weight. Try to maintain a healthy weight. Being overweight or obese puts a strain on your liver. When trying to lose weight, do so gradually, aim for about two pounds per week. Extreme calorie restriction and fad diets are harmful to your liver.

Get Enough Sleep. Sleep is essential for the repair and restoration of all body systems, including the liver. Nighttime is the prime time for the liver to do its restorative functions. Sleep needs vary depending on the individual, but most people need a minimum of 7-8 hours of sleep per night for optimum health.

Control Your Diabetes. If you have diabetes it is essential that you keep tight control over your insulin and glucose levels.

Reduce Stress. Stress is not just taxing to the mind—it has a negative effect on the entire body. The release of stress hormones, including cortisol, can be disruptive to the body's natural rhythms. Chronic stress has been linked to an increase abdominal fat, which is extremely harmful to internal organs, including the liver.

Exercise. Aerobic exercise is beneficial in fighting fatty liver disease. Exercise uses up the excess glucose in your system and makes it easier on the liver to process.

Herbs and Supplements to Support Liver Health

Herbs

Herbs are plants that have compounds that can benefit the body when taken in moderation. Some herbs help relieve inflammation and can reduce the harmful effects of various toxins. Herbs can also be used to promote healthy liver regeneration.

Milk Thistle

This is one of the oldest and most-used herbs for liver-related problems. Thistle milk (*Silybum marianum*) is a herb that gets its name due to the white liquid that is produced when the leaves are crushed. It is known for its anti-inflammatory and antioxidant effects. It helps in detoxification and helps the liver repair and regenerate. In addition, it protects the liver from damage by free radicals. Milk thistle is the most studied and recommended herb for liver health. It is available in capsules or as an extract and is often a key ingredient in many liver tonic pills. Also known as silymarin.

Turmeric

This spice is widely used in cooking and is generally considered safe. It is a natural antioxidant and an anti-inflammatory agent that helps the liver restore itself. It also helps remove the unwanted fat that accumulates in the liver over time. It can be taken in capsule form as well as used in cooking. Also known as curcumin.

Dandelion

The roots, leaves, and flowers of this plant make excellent medicine, not only for the liver, but for the entire gastrointestinal tract. Apart from acting as a direct antioxidant for the liver, dandelion root serves as a mild laxative and helps relieve stomachaches. It can be used in teas and is a natural liver decongestant and helps to restore hepatic function and improve bile production.

Golden Seal

This herb is a wonderful remedy not only for a fatty liver but also various other ailments. It can safely be consumed on a regular basis and is a good lubricating agent that acts as a natural purifier and detoxifying agent. It is also thought to help ward of infections.

Burdock

Used as a blood purifier in Ayurvedic medicine. It stimulates the flow of bile and helps to restore damaged cells.

Ginseng

This is considered by some to be a miracle cure for reduction of fat and cholesterol, not only from the liver, but from the entire body. It is also thought to help lower blood pressure. It is also an antioxidant.

Gentian Root

This herb works to promote liver function and helps in restoring a normal liver. Helps stop liver disease progression.

Ginger

This culinary herb contains a substance called gingerol. Gingerol protects the liver from oxidative stress and helps to strengthen liver recovery.

Cascara Sagrada

This herb enhances liver function, acts as a mild laxative, and also helps in digestion. It stimulates secretion of liver enzymes and bile and inhibits the formation of gallstones.

Green Tea

Green tea is a detoxifying agent. The antioxidants in the tea help to detoxify blood and help control cholesterol and triglyceride levels. Drinking green tea helps boost and strengthen the immune system.

Chicory Root

This medicinal herb has been used for thousands of years to help cleanse the liver.

Globe Artichoke

Contains substances called caffeylquinic acids that have been shown to help repair and regenerate damaged liver cells. Can be taken in capsule form.

Vitamins and Other Supplements

In addition to the above herbs, there are other substances that have been shown to help and protect the liver.

Glutathione

Glutathione, called by some the mother of all antioxidants, is perhaps the most important detoxifier of all. The body produces its own supply of glutathione but in conditions of stress—as from a poor diet, alcohol consumption, aging, overuse of medications, infections, and a host of other common conditions—it does not produce enough of this important antioxidant. Glutathione deficiency has been linked to a host of chronic diseases including heart disease, cancer, diabetes, autism, Alzheimer's disease, Parkinson's disease, chronic fatigue syndrome, arthritis, and especially liver disease. In order to boost your production of glutathione consume sulfur-rich foods such as garlic, onions, and cruciferous vegetables. You can also take a supplement called N-acetyl-cysteine (NAC), a precursor to glutathione, which is used in hospitals for liver failure due to Tylenol overdose.

Vitamin E

Vitamin is a powerful anti-inflammatory and antioxidant. It helps reduce inflammation in the liver and bring the levels of liver enzymes to a normal range.

Vitamin D

This fat-soluble vitamin is stored in the liver. A lack of vitamin D has been linked to poor liver health and to the risk of obesity.

N-Acetyl-l-Cysteine (NAC)

This is an important substance that helps in the formation of glutathione which reduces the oxidative stress throughout the body. NAC is an antioxidant and helps reduce stress on the liver.

Vitamin C

Vitamin C, another powerful antioxidant, has been shown in research to lower the levels of low-density lipoproteins (LDL), the "bad" cholesterol, as well as triglycerides in the liver. Also reduces inflammation.

Alpha Lipoic Acid (ALA)

This is a fatty acid that is readily absorbed in the gut. It converts glucose into energy. It has been shown to help with the fatigue that is commonly associated with a poorly functioning liver.

Vitamin B3 (Niacin)

Niacin has numerous health benefits including conversion of glucose to energy, fat metabolism, and improved liver function. Niacin is best obtained from dietary sources because in large amounts it can damage the liver.

Natural Liver Flush Cleanse

Doing a 7-day natural liver flush is a great way to jump start your weight loss, improve your health, and help get your liver back to peak functioning.

This simple, gentle 7-day plan will have you looking and feeling your best. After completing the weeklong program you should notice significant benefits including clearer skin, reduced abdominal fat and bloating, better sleep, and increased energy. Many people say that after completing a natural liver cleanse they feel years younger.

The purpose of the liver flush is to decongest the bile ducts and help breakdown and eliminate any gallstones that have formed in the gall bladder. This is a pain-free process that will leave your liver functioning better than ever and make you feel healthier than you have in years.

It is helpful to do this cleanse 3-4 times a year in order to maintain optimal liver, gallbladder, and colon health.

Caution: If you have a chronic illness or symptoms of liver disease or failure check with your health care practitioner before embarking on this program. Do not do the liver flush cleanse if you are ill, have a fever, or are suffering from a cold. The liver flush cleanse is not recommended for women who are pregnant or nursing, or for children.

Mechanics and Overview of the Liver Flush Cleanse

The basic idea behind the liver flush is not complicated. It is designed to cleanse the liver of accumulated substances, especially gallstones, which are hindering the liver from its optimal functioning. Years of built-up toxicities will be flushed away, leaving your liver better able to handle its important job of removing toxins from your body.

The main ingredients that are the cornerstones of the liver flush cleanse are:

- Oil—preferably virgin olive oil
- Citrus—lemons, grapefruits, and oranges
- Epsom salt
- Malic acid—found in apples

The 7-day program is broken up into 3 phases. The first phase, on days 1-5, involves preparing the body by cleaning up the diet and drinking juices containing malic acid. The sixth day of the program is a juice fast to help clear the body of any remaining toxicities. Finally, on the evening of the six day and into the seventh day, is the actual overnight liver flush. It involves consuming a combination of Epsom salt, lemon juice, and olive oil.

Each of these three phases will be detailed in the coming pages.

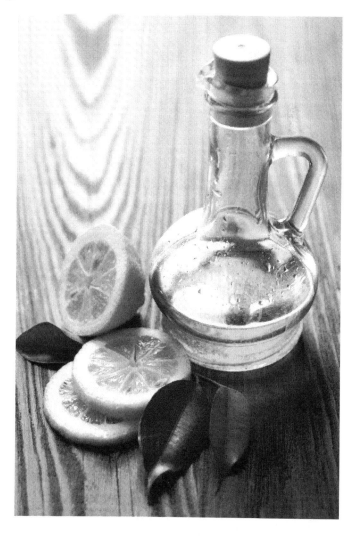

Preparation for Liver Flush

In order to complete the 7-day program successfully you are going to need to have a number of items on hand. The majority should be readily available in your local grocery store, and in fact, you may already have them in your pantry.

GROCERY ITEMS

*Leafy green vegetables—The first 5 days of the liver cleanse rely heavily on fresh, preferably organic, fruits and vegetables. These vegetables will help prepare the liver and body for the overnight liver detox on the final day. They have a powerful protective effect on the liver and will support the production of bile. You can eat them raw (in salads), cooked (steamed, in soups, etc.), or use them in green smoothies. Some to have on hand include kale, spinach, arugula, mustard greens, chicory, and dandelion greens.

*Apple juice—During the first 6 days, you will be drinking rather large quantities (32 ounces) of apple juice. It is the malic acid contained in the apple juice that is going to help soften and break down the gallstones, making them easier to flush. In addition, malic acid is a known metal chelator; it is able to bind with toxic heavy metals that have accumulated in the body and help flush them out. You can either buy the apples and juice them yourself or you can just purchase the juice. Be sure to get 100%, organic apple juice.

If you prefer, you can substitute part or all of the apple juice with either cherry juice or cranberry juice. Be sure to buy 100% juice and then dilute it yourself. If you have candida, diabetes, or are overweight, then diluted cranberry juice may be your best option. Dilute one part juice with two parts filtered water.

* **Lemons, limes, and grapefruit**—These citrus fruits are high in both vitamin C and antioxidants. They boost the production of liver detox enzymes and aid in the removal of carcinogens and other toxins. You will be consuming a daily glass of lemon and water throughout the 7 days. In addition, you will be using either lemon or grapefruit juice mixed with oil during the overnight flush.

* **Cruciferous vegetables**—These types of vegetables boost the enzyme production in the liver. Stock up on broccoli and cauliflower.

* **Extra-virgin olive oil**—This cold-pressed oil is a vital ingredient in the final phase of the liver cleanse. The lipids in the oil help to absorb toxins and also serve as a necessary lubricant to make excretion of the gallstones a smooth and painless procedure. Be sure that you

purchase extra-virgin olive oil. Possible substitutes include other cold-pressed oils such as flaxseed, hemp, grape seed, or sunflower.

* **Epsom salt**—The magnesium sulphate found in Epsom salt is critical to the liver flush.

* **Ginger root**—Ginger is a wonderful antioxidant and also helps to lower triglycerides. Several studies have indicated ginger as a possible treatment for fatty liver disease. Ginger can be taken as a tea and also can be freshly grated into dressings, soups, or smoothies. Also try grating a little ginger into your morning glass of lemon and water for a little extra zing.

* **Garlic**—Garlic has numerous benefits for the liver, including being a great source of both selenium and allicin, two compounds that aid in liver cleansing.

* **Walnuts**—Walnuts are high in omega-3 fatty acids, glutathione, and arginine, all of which support and aid the liver's cleansing functions.

* **Green and herbal teas**—Throughout the cleanse you will be sipping on various teas. Green tea contains catechins, a substance that assists liver function. Dandelion root tea is another tea known for its liver-benefitting properties.

* **Turmeric**—If the liver had a favorite spice, this would be it.

* **Other vegetables**—In addition to those mentioned above, the following will help cleanse and support your liver: avocado, artichoke, asparagus, cabbage, and Brussels sprouts. Try to incorporate as many as possible into your 7-day meal plan.

* **Whole grains and alternative grains**—To decrease the toxic load on your liver, you will be cutting out all processed foods and white flour. While the majority of the foods you eat during the week should be fruits and vegetables, it is fine to incorporate a moderate amount of whole grains into your diet. Choose whole wheat, oats, quinoa, and brown rice.

TOOLS AND OTHER SUPPLIES

A few other basic supplies will be needed:

***Glass bottles or jars with lids**—For storing your salt and water mixture as well as your oil and citrus blend.

***Blender**—For making smoothies.

***Juicer**—This is not an absolute requirement, but it is nice to have for juicing your own fruits and vegetables.

ADDITIONAL PREPARATIONS

To make the process of cleansing the liver easier and to reduce any side effects from detoxification (such as headaches, lightheadedness, aches, diarrhea) it is best to ease into it slowly by avoiding the consumption of alcohol, animals products (meat and dairy), processed foods, caffeine, and fried foods for several days leading up to the actual liver cleanse. Also, try not to take any medications or supplements in the days leading up to the cleanse, aside from medically necessary prescription medications. This is because these substances put extra stress on the liver and we want it to be able to devote all of its resources to the cleanse.

TIMING OF THE CLEANSE

It is best to time the final part of the liver flush for a period of time when you do not have a lot of work or responsibilities to attend to and will have enough time for rest and relaxation, such as over a weekend.

Rules to Follow on the 7-Day Cleanse

For best results during the cleanse, follow these guidelines:

Avoid eating within 3 hours of bedtime. This will allow your digestive system to be clear so that your liver can focus on detoxification while you sleep.

Avoid alcohol and caffeine. These are taxing substances for the liver and will force the liver to expend its energy on clearing them out.

Use a sauna. If available, taking a daily sauna during this week will enhance your detox efforts. The skin is a major detoxification organ and toxins will be released in your sweat.

Take a bath with Epsom salts. A relaxing Epsom salt bath is very beneficial during your detoxification. The magnesium and sulfates in the salts will get absorbed through the skin and aid in the flushing of toxins. Magnesium aids in the production of bile. Take a soak nightly as part of your evening routine.

Body brushing. Using a loofah or firm, natural fiber brush, brush your skin with circular strokes, starting from the feet and working your way up toward your arms and shoulders. Avoid your face, neck, and spots that are irritated with rash or cuts. Doing this will improve your circulation and help to release toxins through the skin. Follow with a shower.

Practice yoga and meditation. Being under stress releases hormones, like cortisol, that also tax the liver and slow its functioning. Make time every day to de-stress. Fifteen minutes of sitting quietly in meditation or doing yoga will help settle your mind and relax your body.

The 7-Day Plan

During days 1-5 of the cleanse, you will be preparing your body for the actual liver flush on the sixth and seventh days. Foods to eat during this time include berries (blueberries, raspberries, blackberries, strawberries, cranberries), apples, cherries, citrus fruit (lemons grapefruit, orange), dark green vegetables (spinach, kale, collard greens, romaine lettuce), avocado, cruciferous vegetables (broccoli, Brussels sprouts, cabbage), garlic, fennel, shitake mushrooms, spices (turmeric, cinnamon), walnuts, and fermented foods such as kefir, kambucha, and sauerkraut.

In addition, each day you will need to consume 32 ounces (4 glasses) of pure organic apple juice (or substitute with part or all cherry or cranberry juice). Set this aside in the morning and sip on it throughout each day.

What follows is a suggested menu plan. Feel free to mix and match based on your specific needs and preferences.

Day 1:

Before breakfast: First thing in the morning, drink an 8 oz. glass of room temperature filtered water with the juice of 1/2 a lemon squeezed into it. *Optional:* Grate in fresh ginger.

Breakfast: Fruit smoothie*—Combine your choice of blueberries, strawberries, raspberries with banana and either kefir milk, rice milk, almond milk, or freshly squeezed orange juice. *Optional:* Add a scoop of protein powder.

Mid-morning snack: Celery sticks dipped in hummus.

Lunch: Spinach salad, glass of water with lemon.

Afternoon: Simple guacamole with carrot sticks. Cup of green tea.

Dinner: Lentil soup, baked sweet potato.

Before bed: Drink a soothing detox tea such as milk thistle, burdock, or dandelion root.

Throughout the day: In addition to the apple, cherry, or cranberry juice, sip on water with fresh lemon, herbal tea, and green tea in unlimited quantities. Additionally, snack on raw veggies in unlimited quantities.

Day 2:

Before breakfast: First thing in the morning, drink an 8 oz. glass of room temperature filtered water with the juice of 1/2 a lemon squeezed into it. *Optional:* Grate in fresh ginger.

Breakfast: Oatmeal topped with fresh berries and sprinkled with walnuts.

Mid-morning snack: Pear or apple with almond butter.

Lunch: Spring mix salad topped with avocado, tomatoes, and shredded carrots. Lemon-turmeric-balsamic dressing.

Afternoon: Green smoothie.

Dinner: Veggie stir fry over brown rice—Your choice of veggies: broccoli, carrots, sprouts, leeks, mushrooms, pea pods.

Before bed: Drink a soothing detox tea such as milk thistle, burdock, or dandelion root.

Throughout the day: In addition to the apple, cherry, or cranberry juice, sip on water with fresh lemon, herbal tea, and green tea in unlimited quantities. Additionally, snack on raw veggies in unlimited quantities.

Day 3:

Before breakfast: First thing in the morning, drink an 8 oz. glass of room temperature filtered water with the juice of 1/2 a lemon squeezed into it. *Optional:* Grate in fresh ginger.

Breakfast: Mango and banana smoothie.

Mid-morning snack: Air-popped popcorn seasoned with sea salt and pepper.

Lunch: Taco salad—Romaine lettuce topped with black beans, diced tomato, red onion, and avocado. Glass of water with lemon.

Afternoon: Handful of almonds or walnuts. Cup of green tea.

Dinner: Vegetable curry—Combine sweet potatoes, cauliflower, chickpeas, and carrots in casserole dish. Add can of coconut milk, 1 cup of water, and curry spices (cumin, tumeric, cayenne). Bake in oven until vegetables are tender.

Before bed: Drink a soothing detox tea such as milk thistle, burdock, or dandelion root.

Throughout the day: In addition to the apple, cherry, or cranberry juice, sip on water with fresh lemon, herbal tea, and green tea in unlimited quantities. Additionally, snack on raw veggies in unlimited quantities.

Day 4:

Before breakfast: First thing in the morning, drink an 8 oz. glass of room temperature filtered water with the juice of 1/2 a lemon squeezed into it. *Optional:* Grate in fresh ginger.

Breakfast: Slice of whole-grain bread topped with 1 tablespoon peanut butter and 1/2 a banana or apple slices.

Mid-morning snack: Raw veggies with hummus.

Lunch: Beet salad

Afternoon: Chai cacao shake

Dinner: Steamed salmon with lemon over quinoa. Steamed broccoli.

Before bed: Drink a soothing detox tea such as milk thistle, burdock, or dandelion root.

Throughout the day: In addition to the apple, cherry, or cranberry juice, sip on water with fresh lemon, herbal tea, and green tea in unlimited quantities. Additionally, snack on raw veggies in unlimited quantities.

Day 5:

Before breakfast: First thing in the morning, drink an 8 oz. glass of room temperature filtered water with the juice of 1/2 a lemon squeezed into it. *Optional:* Grate in fresh ginger.

Breakfast: Fruit smoothie*—Combine your choice of blueberries, strawberries, raspberries with banana and either kefir milk, rice milk, almond milk, or freshly squeezed orange juice. Optional: Add a scoop of protein powder.

Mid-morning snack: Celery sticks dipped in hummus. Glass of apple juice.

Lunch: Hearty salad topped with tuna

Afternoon: Brown rice cakes topped with nut butter

Dinner: Black and red bean chili.

Before bed: Drink a soothing detox tea such as milk thistle, burdock, or dandelion root.

Throughout the day: In addition to the apple, cherry, or cranberry juice, sip on water with fresh lemon, herbal tea, and green tea in unlimited quantities. Additionally, snack on raw veggies in unlimited quantities.

Days 6-7: The sixth day calls for a liquids-only fast up until you start the actual overnight liver flush.

Breakfast: Fruit smoothie

Lunch: Green smoothie

In addition, you will need to drink all of your apple juice (or cherry or cranberry) before 2 p.m. Do not consume any food or juices after 2 p.m. on the sixth day. You can, however, drink water if you are thirsty.

THE OVERNIGHT LIVER FLUSH

Now it is time for the actual liver flush. The past six days have prepared your liver and the rest of your body and so you should not experience any detrimental side effects.

To do the flush you will need:

- 4 tablespoons of Epsom salt
- 3 cups of water
- 1/2 cup of extra-virgin olive oil
- 2 grapefruits, lemons, or oranges

In one of your jars or bottles with a lid, mix the 4 tablespoons of Epsom salt with the 3 cups of water. Put the cover on, and shake until the salt is dissolved in the water. You will need to divide it into four equal portions. Do not refrigerate.

At **6 p.m.**, drink your first serving of the Epsom salt and water mixture. It will not taste great, so just hold your nose and get it down as quickly as possible.

Two hours later, at **8 p.m.**, drink your second serving of the salt and water solution.

Now it is time to prepare the oil and citrus solution. Squeeze out a 1/2 cup (4 ounces) of your chosen citrus juice (grapefruit, lemon, or orange) into a jar. Pour in 1/2 cup of extra-virgin olive oil. Cover tightly and shake well.

At **10 p.m.** drink down the oil and citrus mixture. Again, this is not going to taste great. You may even feel like vomiting. Just take deep breathes and try to relax. Walk around a little if it helps. If you absolutely cannot get the mixture down, try adding a little honey to it.

Once you've got the oil mixture down, go to bed. Lie on your back and try not to get up, except if you need to use the bathroom. Do not drink anything else for at least 2 hours.

At **6 a.m.** wake up and drink the third portion of your water and salt solution. Do not go back to bed. At this point, you want to remain upright, doing light activities, to help the movement of noxious substances out of your liver and colon.

At **8 a.m.** it is time to drink the last of your water and salt. You will want to stay close to the bathroom for the rest of the morning. You may experience diarrhea for the rest of the day. If you look into the bowl, you will likely see a number of gallstone being expelled. They can range in color from shades of green, to browns, and even black. Do not be alarmed, this is normal and expected.

Wait a couple of hours after your last glass of salt water before consuming anything else. You can then resume eating normally, although it is best to eat lightly for the rest of the day. Start slowly, with a piece of fruit or some raw vegetables.

That completes your 7-day liver flush cleanse.

Follow-up and Expected Results

A common occurrence during a detoxification program such as this one is what is known as a "healing crisis." Many people find that during the first few days of following a detox diet they feel somewhat unwell with symptoms that may include headache, body aches, fatigue, cramps, nausea, lightheadedness, and weakness. This is due to the withdrawal effects from substances such as sugar, alcohol, and caffeine. In addition, as you detox, your organs are releasing many pent-up toxins into your bloodstream, which can also lead to the above symptoms. These symptoms are temporary, usually lasting only about 48 hours. The best way to combat these symptoms is by drinking lots of fluids to help flush the toxins out of your system. If symptoms are severe, you may need to have more frequent snacks, increase your intake of protein and healthy fats, and make sure you are getting an adequate amount of rest. After several days, your symptoms should clear and you will find yourself feeling better and more energized than ever.

Results from the 7-day liver cleanse flush vary from person to person, but the majority of people find that they lose weight (typically 5-8 pounds), sleep better, have decreased joint and muscle pain, have smoother and clearer skin, and feel more energetic.

Conclusion

Now that you have completed the 7-day liver flush and cleanse it is important to continue your healthy habits. Do not go back to your normal routine. Instead, try to continue the healthy habits started here for increased liver and overall health.

The liver is one of the most important organs in the body and its proper functioning is vital to our overall feelings of health and well-being. Take care of your liver and it will take care of you.

Resources and References

- http://www.patient.co.uk/health/non-alcoholic-fatty-liver-disease
- http://www.thenutritiondr.com/low-carbohydrate-carb-dietbody-fatweight-lossglycemic-indexglycemic-loadglucose-tolerance-test-curve-diabetes/
- http://healthyeating.sfgate.com/sugars-transported-liver-convert-glucose-2090.html
- http://www.liverdoctor.com/liver/fatty-liver/
- http://www.naturalnews.com/036466_NAFLD_natural_treatment.html#
- http://www.betterhealth.vic.gov.au/bhcv2/bhcarticles.nsf/pages/Liver_disease_fatty_liver_disease
- http://fattylivercured.com/
- http://drhyman.com/blog/2013/09/26/fatty-liver-90-million-americans/#close
- http://www.sciencedirect.com/science/article/pii/S0891584907008416
- http://www.ivillage.ca/health/diet/9-most-popular-cleanse-and-detox-diets-SR
- http://www.webmd.com/diet/features/detox-diets-cleansing-body

- http://life.gaiam.com/article/10-ways-detoxify-your-body
- http://www.diseaseproof.com/archives/hurtful-food-saturated-fat-vs-polyunsaturated-fat.html
- http://www.mayoclinic.org/diseases-conditions/nonalcoholic-fatty-liver-disease/basics/lifestyle-home-remedies/con-20027761
- http://www.mayoclinic.org/diseases-conditions/nonalcoholic-fatty-liver-disease/basics/alternative-medicine/con-20027761
- http://www.healthkart.com/resources/reverse-fatty-liver-symptoms-naturally/#.U6mminKSxHE
- http://www.newportnaturalhealth.com/2012/04/show-your-liver-some-love/
- http://www.wellnessresources.com/weight/articles/unclog_your_liver_lose_your_abdominal_fat_l eptin_diet_weight_loss_challenge/

From the Author

Thank you for reading *The Natural Liver Flush: 7-Day Liver Cleanse Diet to Revitalize Your Health, Detox Your Body, and Reverse Fatty Liver.* I sincerely hope that you found this book informative and helpful.

It would be greatly appreciated if you could take a few moments to share your opinion and post a review for this book on Amazon or other retailer where you purchased this book. Your positive review helps us to reach other readers and provides valuable feedback with which we can improve future books.

Thank you!

49235186R00039

Made in the USA
Middletown, DE
10 October 2017